Wars Waged Under the Microscope

The War Against Cancer

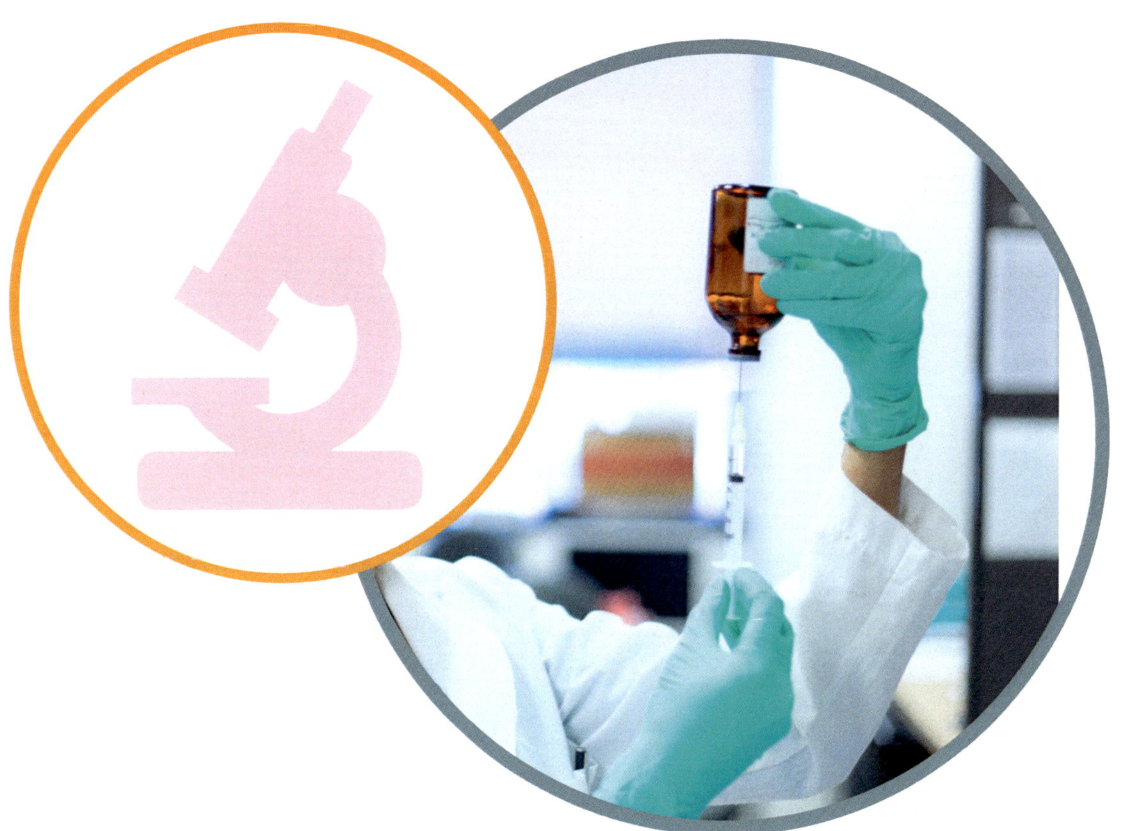

Sarah Eason

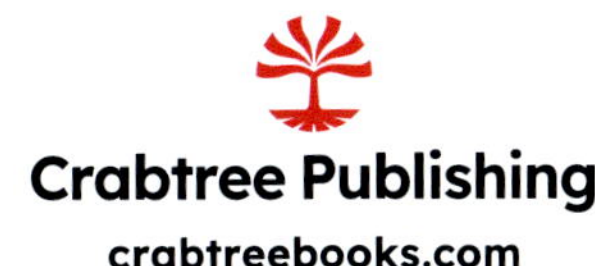

Crabtree Publishing

crabtreebooks.com 800-387-7650

Published in Canada
Crabtree Publishing
616 Welland Avenue
St. Catharines, Ontario
L2M 5V6

Published in the United States
Crabtree Publishing
347 Fifth Avenue
Suite 1402-145
New York, NY 10016

Author: Sarah Eason
Editors: Jennifer Sanderson and Ellen Rodger
Editorial director: Kathy Middleton
Design: Simon Borrough
Cover design and additional artwork: Katherine Kantor
Photo research: Rachel Blount
Proofreader: Wendy Scavuzzo
Production coordinator and
Prepress technician: Ken Wright
Print coordinator: Katherine Kantor
Consultant: David Hawksett
Produced for Crabtree Publishing by Calcium Creative Ltd

Printed in Canada/082024/CPC20240819

Library and Archives Canada Cataloguing in Publication
Title: The war against cancer / Sarah Eason.
Names: Eason, Sarah, author.
Description: Series statement: Wars waged under the microscope | Includes bibliographical references and index.
Identifiers: Canadiana (print) 20210189002 | Canadiana (ebook) 20210189010 | ISBN 9781427151278 (hardcover) | ISBN 9781427151353 (softcover) | ISBN 9781427151438 (HTML) | ISBN 9781427151513 (EPUB)
Subjects: LCSH: Cancer—Juvenile literature. | LCSH: Cancer—Treatment—Juvenile literature. | LCSH: Cancer—Prevention—Juvenile literature.
Classification: LCC RC264 .E27 2022 | DDC j614.5/999—dc23

Photo Credits

Cover: All images Shutterstock

Inside: Shutterstock: pp. 28-29; Andreonegin: p. 13; Maliutina Anna: p. 11; AshTproductions: p. 27; Elnur: p. 18; Excellent Dream: p. 8; Gorodenkoff: p. 24; Image Point Fr: p. 17; Inbevel: p. 6; Jarva Jar: p. 10; Lightspring: p. 26; David A Litman: p. 9; Komsan Loonprom: p. 25; Ramniklal Modi: p. 21; Monkey Business Images: p. 19; Sandra Morante: p. 23; Tyler Olson: p. 16; Saikat Paul: p. 22; Peakstock: p. 15; Arjen de Ruiter: p. 20; SciePro: pp. 14-15; Shebeko: pp. 4, 31; TravnikovStudio: p. 12; Wikimedia Commons: Photograph by J. C. Schaarwächter, 1891/ Wellcome Images: p. 7; Wellcome Images: p. 5.

Hardcover 978-1-4271-5127-8
Paperback 978-1-4271-5135-3
Ebook (pdf) 978-1-4271-5143-8
Epub 978-1-4271-5151-3

Library of Congress Cataloging-in-Publication Data
Names: Eason, Sarah, author.
Title: The war against cancer / Sarah Eason.
Description: New York, NY : Crabtree Publishing Company, [2022] | Series: Wars waged under the microscope | Includes index.
Identifiers: LCCN 2021016650 (print) | LCCN 2021016651 (ebook) | ISBN 9781427151278 (hardcover) | ISBN 9781427151353 (paperback) | ISBN 9781427151438 (ebook) | ISBN 9781427151513 (epub)
Subjects: LCSH: Cancer--Juvenile literature. | Cancer--Treatment--Juvenile literature. | Cancer--Prevention--Juvenile literature.
Classification: LCC RC264 .E27 2022 (print) | LCC RC264 (ebook) | DDC 616.99/4--dc23
LC record available at https://lccn.loc.gov/2021016650
LC ebook record available at https://lccn.loc.gov/2021016651

Contents

The Enemy 4
The Battle Begins 6
An Invisible Threat 8
Signs of Attack 10
Targeting Skin Cancer 12
Case Study: Rare Skin Cancer Study 13
Studying the Enemy 14
Armed with Medicine 16
Vital Testing 18
Case Study: Groundbreaking Cancer Trial 19
A Worldwide Fight 20
Enemy Education 22
Case Study: Knowledge Is Power 23
New Weapons 24
Future Warfare 26
Timeline 28
Glossary 30
Learning More 31
Index and About the Author 32

The Enemy

Cancer is often feared as a deadly disease. However, medical science is constantly searching for solutions in its fight against this tiny enemy. Many breakthroughs in recent years have meant the disease—once always a killer—can now be treated and often cured. None of these breakthroughs would have been possible were it not for powerful microscopes. These tools have allowed scientists to identify and study what would otherwise be impossible to see with the naked eye.

What Is Cancer?

All living things are made up of tiny cells that can be seen only under a microscope. The human body has about 30 trillion cells. "Cancer" is a word given to more than 200 different diseases that are caused when cells in the body start to grow abnormally. Some of the many types of cancer include skin cancer, breast cancer, **bowel** cancer, and lung cancer.

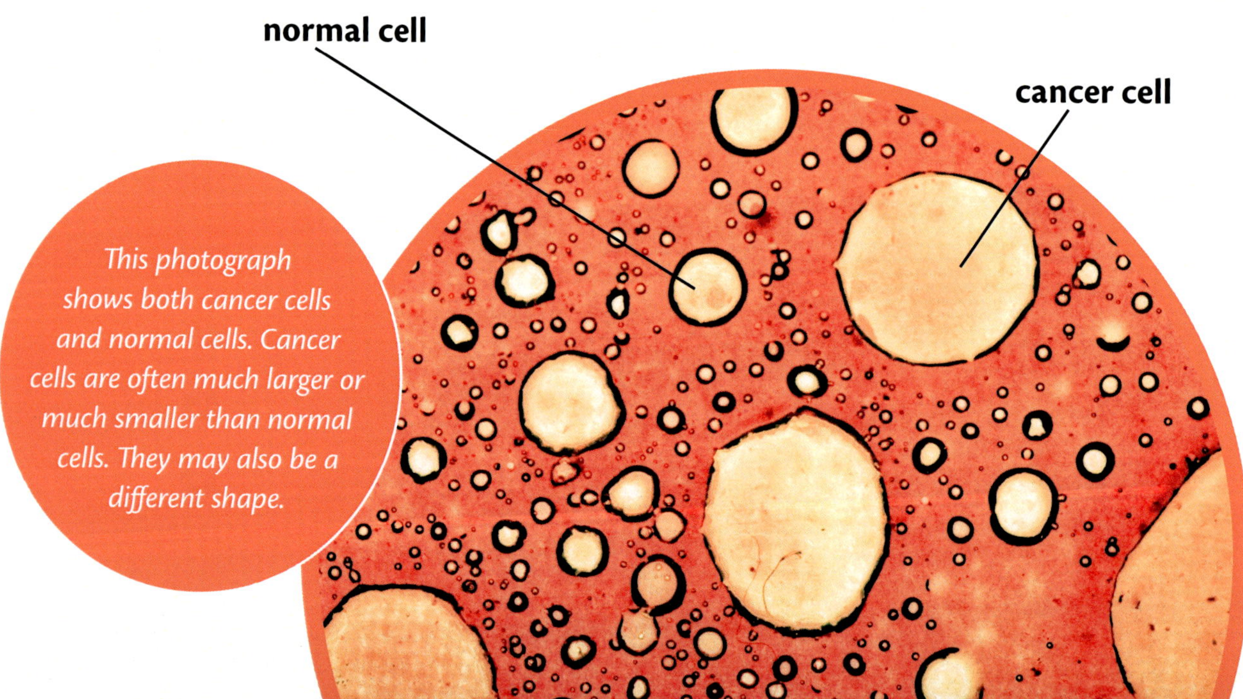

This photograph shows both cancer cells and normal cells. Cancer cells are often much larger or much smaller than normal cells. They may also be a different shape.

The Story of Cancer

The first recorded, or written down, cases of cancer date back to ancient Egyptian times. The Greeks later identified and gave the disease the name "*carcinos*," which the Romans then translated to "cancer." However, it was not until many centuries after the Romans that people discovered cancer takes place inside the body at a **cellular** level, hidden from the naked eye.

The journey to discovering cells and cancer cells began in the 1590s in Holland, when a man named Hans Janssen and his son Zacharias built a device that could magnify objects, or make them bigger. The Janssen discovery then led to the invention of the microscope, which allowed scientists to study blood and **tissue**, and figure out how they worked. In 1665, English **physicist** Robert Hooke used the microscope to identify curved structures in human tissue. To Hooke, they looked like the rooms monks lived in, known as cells, and he named the structures "cells."

Hooke studied cells using an early microscope like this one. Modern-day microscopes are so advanced that some can cut tissue with a ***laser****, to reveal cancer cells within it.*

"By the help of microscopes, there is nothing so small, as to escape our inquiry; hence there is a new visible world discovered to the understanding."

Robert Hooke

The Battle Begins

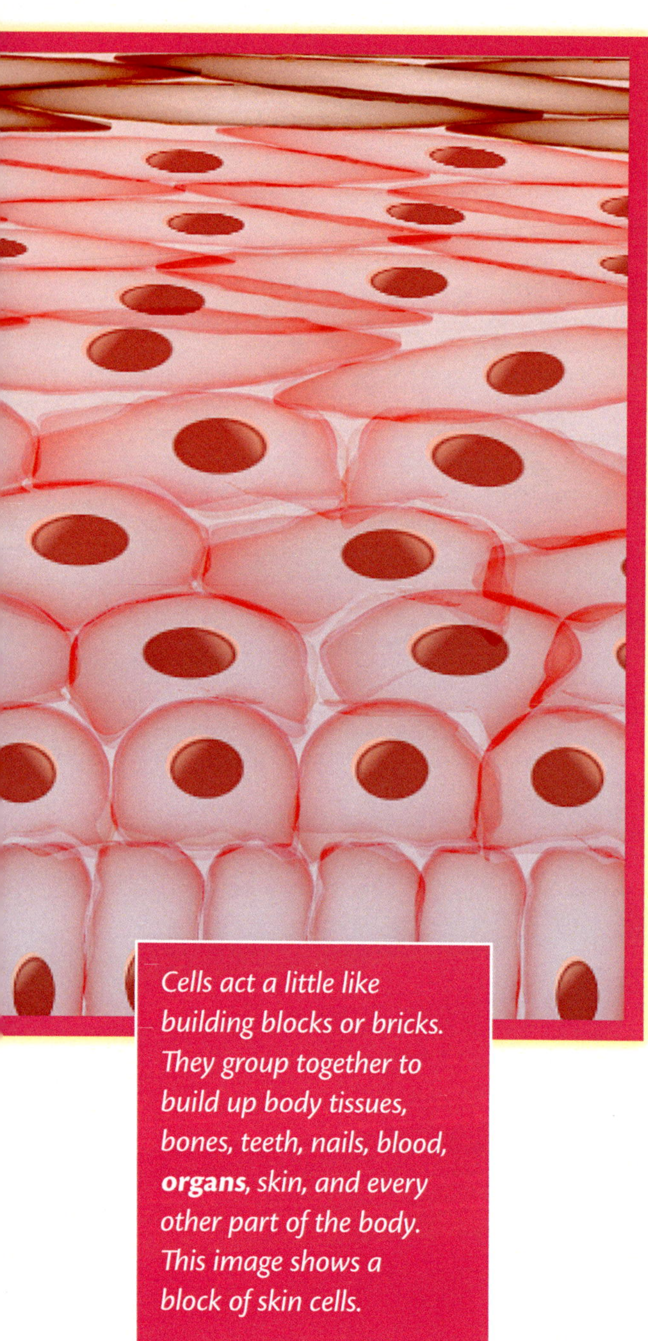

Cells act a little like building blocks or bricks. They group together to build up body tissues, bones, teeth, nails, blood, ***organs****, skin, and every other part of the body. This image shows a block of skin cells.*

In 1839, almost 200 years after Hooke discovered cells, the German scientists Matthias Schleiden and Theodor Schwann came up with the theory that all living things are made up of cells, and that they act as the "building blocks" for all life. This became known as cell theory.

Cells and Cancer

In 1858, the Polish scientist Rudolf Virchow developed cell theory further. He studied cells under the microscope, too, and concluded that all diseases can be traced back to cells. Virchow was the first person to suggest that cancer cells began as healthy cells that then became unhealthy.

Virchow's discoveries forever changed how people investigate and understand cancer. With his realization that all diseases can be traced back to cells, from the late 1800s, scientists began to seriously study diseases and what causes them. This study of diseases and their causes is known as pathology.

Identifying Cancer

As microscopes became more powerful in the 1900s, scientists were able to use them to study cancer cells in far more detail. Since then, scientists and doctors have discovered more and more about how cells work, and what causes cells to become abnormal in different parts of the body. This has enabled them to identify different types of cancer.

Virchow taught medical students in Germany. He was known for being passionate about encouraging his students to use microscopes and think "microscopically" all the time.

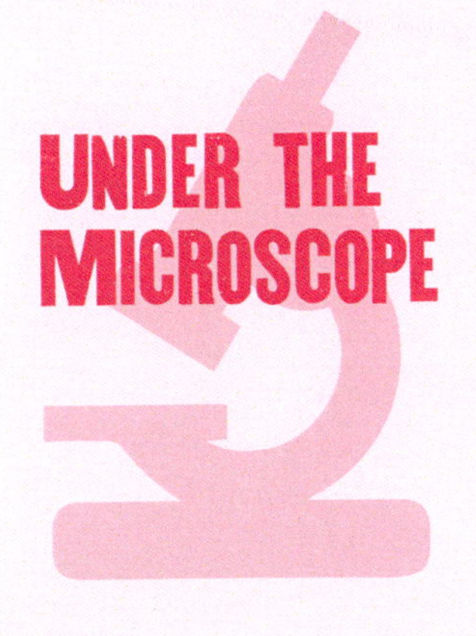

Virchow used **autopsies** to learn more about people's cells and cancer. In 1845, he carried out an autopsy on a 50-year-old woman and discovered an unusually high number of **white blood cells** in her body. He concluded that this was a form of cancer. In 1857, he named the cancer leukemia.

An Invisible Threat

With many cancers, the disease is there before the person realizes they are sick. Unlike some illnesses that have more obvious symptoms, or signs of illness, cancer sometimes shows no signs at all.

Dividing Cells

When a cell is damaged or dies, the body produces new cells by dividing them into two. Some cells, such as skin cells, are dividing all the time, while others, such as brain cells, hardly ever divide. Each cell has a "control center" called the nucleus. Inside the nucleus are **genes** that contain coded messages in the form of **deoxyribonucleic acid (DNA)**. The genes make sure the cells divide and grow normally and perform the job they are supposed to do to keep a body healthy.

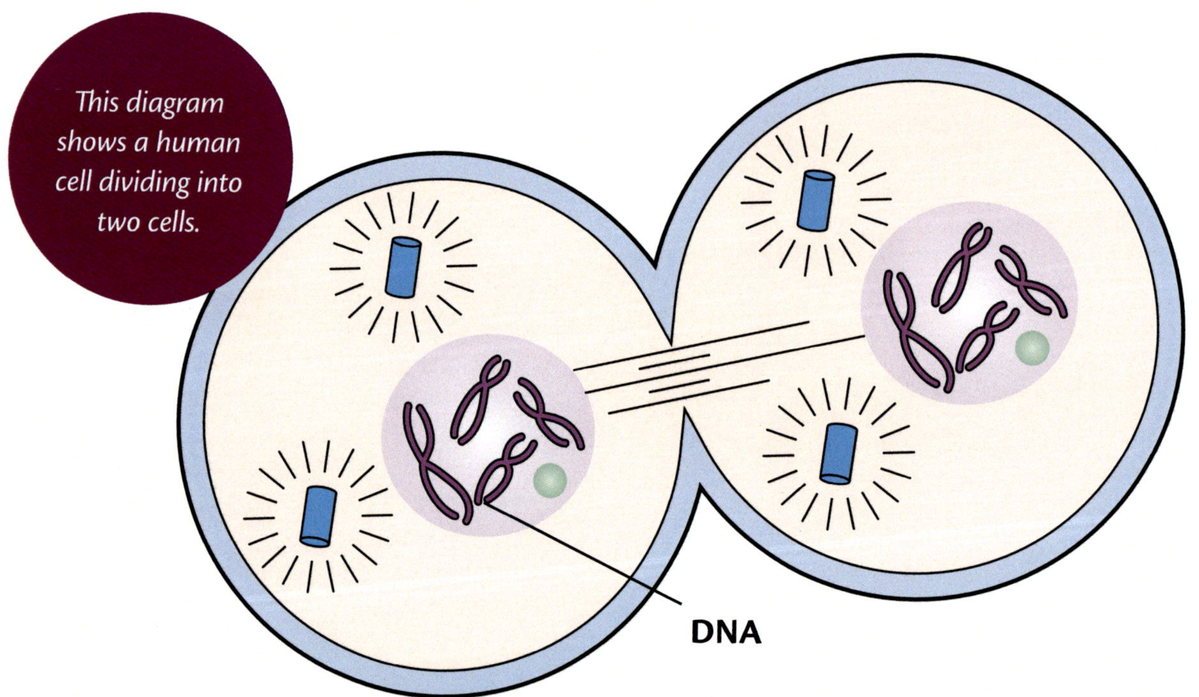

This diagram shows a human cell dividing into two cells.

Hidden Changes

Through microscopy, or studying things under a microscope, scientists have learned a lot about how cells work. When cells divide into two, signals within the cells make sure that a body always has the right type and number of cells. If the signals go wrong because a cell is damaged, it does not divide as it should. The type and number of cells in the body then becomes unbalanced, paving the way for cancer.

Laboratory Checks

Damaged cells multiply too fast and grow too quickly. In some instances, this can cause a **tumor**. However, not all cancers form tumors. A doctor will carry out a biopsy on the tumor to see if it has cancer cells. In a biopsy, the doctor takes a small slice of tissue, known as a sample, from the tumor. The sample is then sent to a laboratory where it is examined under a microscope for cancer cells. This will show whether the tumor is benign or malignant. Benign means it is not cancerous and the cells will not divide and spread to other parts of the body. Malignant means it is cancerous and the cells can divide and spread to other parts of the body.

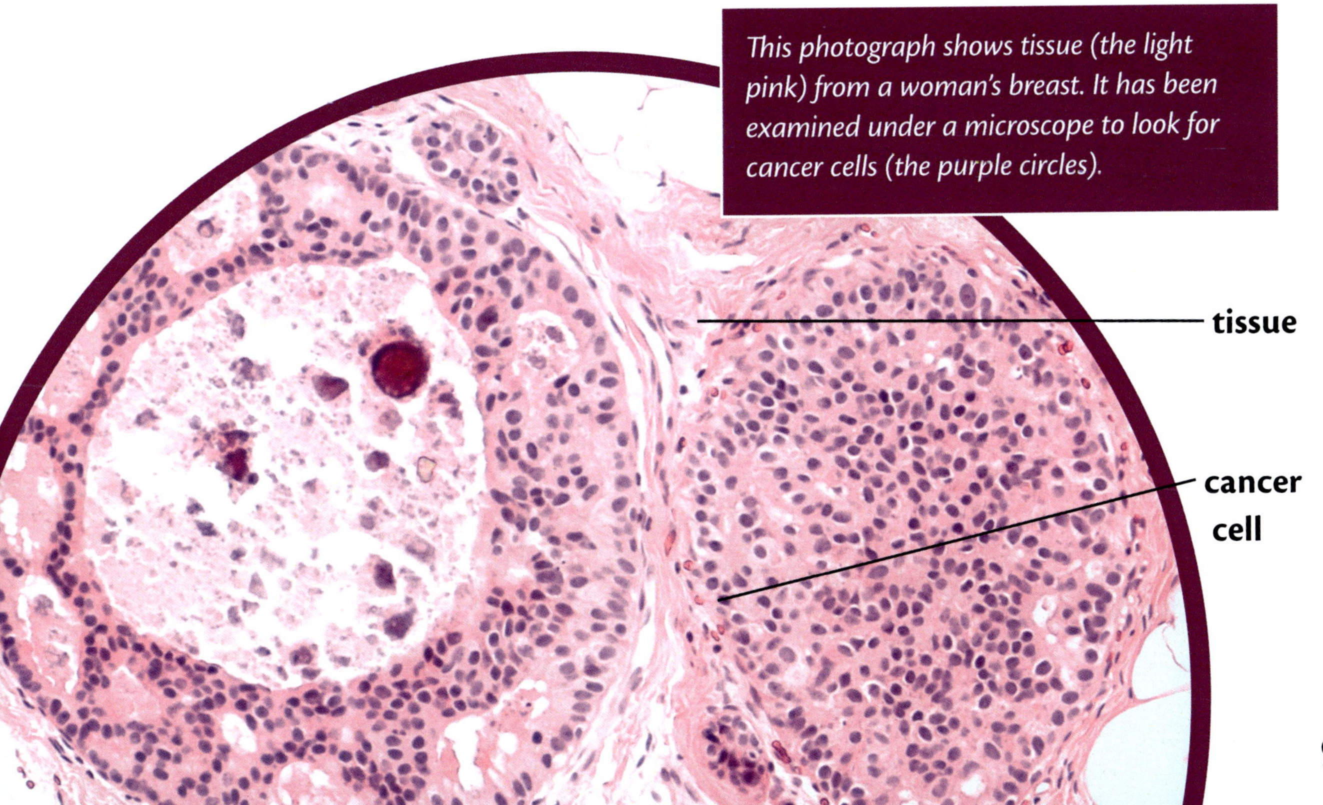

This photograph shows tissue (the light pink) from a woman's breast. It has been examined under a microscope to look for cancer cells (the purple circles).

Signs of Attack

Different cancers damage the body in different ways, depending on where they are located. As we know, all cancer begins in a person's cells, so that is where the war against this disease must be fought—whatever its location in the body.

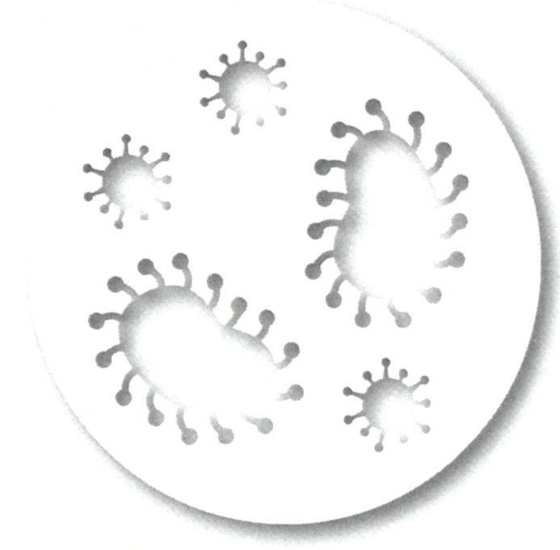

Doctors may use imaging tests such as X-rays to find cancers. X-rays can see through a person's skin and to their bones. X-rays produce images like this one, which shows a person's lungs and the signs of cancer in them.

Many Symptoms

When a group of cancer cells in a tumor starts to grow, this can make the person sick and cause symptoms that include itchiness, redness, muscle aches, pain, weight loss, bleeding, and headaches. These symptoms can also be signs of other illnesses, so finding a cancer and treating it usually begins with a trip to the doctor and a number of tests.

Signs of Leukemia

One of the many types of cancer is leukemia, which is a cancer of the blood and bone marrow. Bone marrow is the spongy tissue found in the spaces inside bones. Leukemia affects white blood cells, which protect the body from infection. In leukemia, abnormal cells flood the blood, leaving no room for normal white blood cells. The person is then open to infection, bleeds easily, and feels tired.

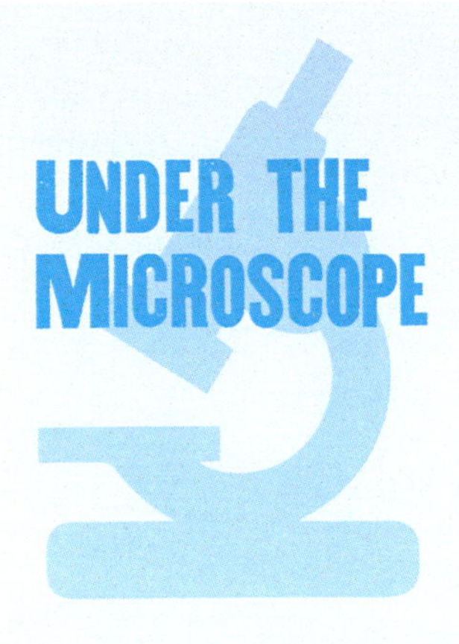

Hematologist-oncologists are doctors who specialize in diagnosing and treating blood diseases, including leukemia. In someone with leukemia, cancerous blood cells are made in bone marrow, so a hematologist-oncologist will take a sample of the patient's bone marrow and examine it for any abnormal cells. There are different types of leukemia, so the specialist will also find out which type a patient has so it can be treated properly. The hematologist-oncologist will shape a patient's treatment plan so that his or her particular type of cancer is targeted and attacked with the most effective methods.

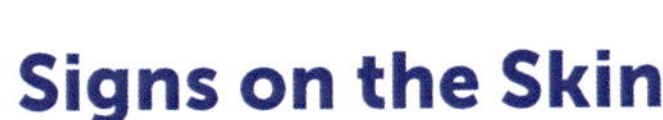

Signs on the Skin

Skin cancer is one of the most common cancers and it is easy to treat if it is caught early enough. Early signs are sores on the skin that will not heal, a reddish patch that may itch or cause no discomfort, **moles** that change shape or color, and unusual changes in the skin. Skin cancers are usually caused by too much exposure to the Sun's harmful **ultraviolet (UV)** rays.

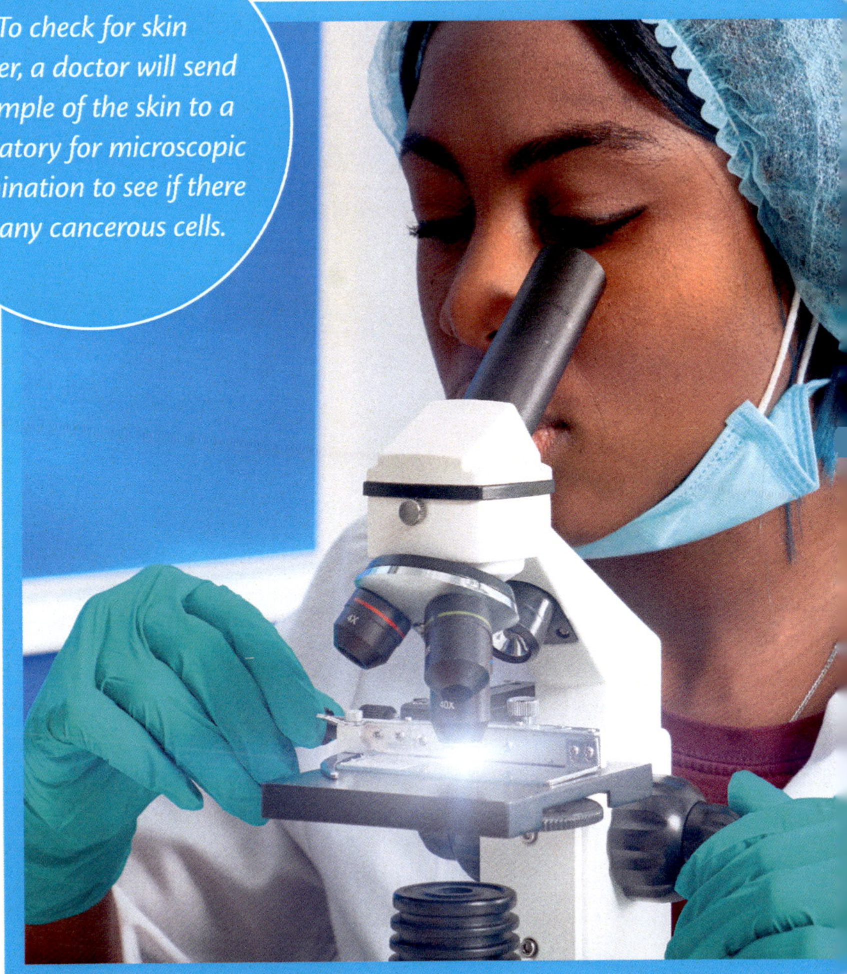

To check for skin cancer, a doctor will send a sample of the skin to a laboratory for microscopic examination to see if there are any cancerous cells.

Targeting Skin Cancer

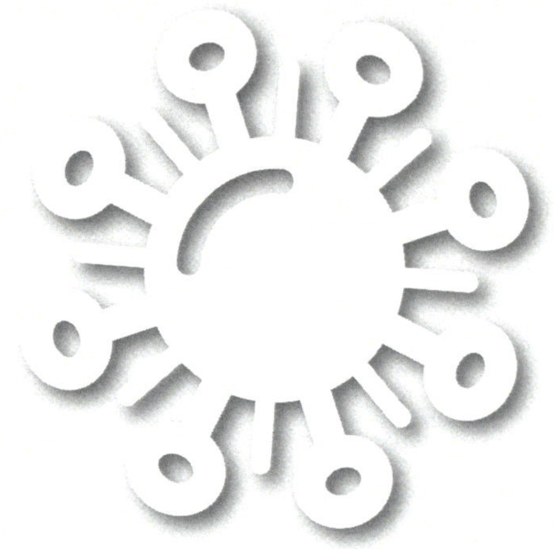

In recent years, scientists and researchers have discovered a lot about skin cancer. They have learned more about how this particular cancer forms, and how to treat it. As with every disease, the best treatment of all is prevention. That is why scientists and governments are trying to make more people aware of skin cancer, and take steps to prevent it.

Battling the Enemy

Through education about skin cancer, most people now know that too much exposure to UV rays damages skin cells, which can lead to cancer. As a result, more people are protecting their skin from the harmful effects of the Sun. Through carefully studying skin cancer, researchers have also been able to create new, more effective treatments for the disease that greatly improve people's chances of recovery.

Part of the battle against skin cancer is to use sunscreen or sunblock to protect the skin from damaging sunlight.

CASE STUDY: RARE SKIN CANCER STUDY

In 2016, researchers in a study announced that there had been a breakthrough in the treatment of malignant melanoma, a skin cancer.

The study was carried out by the Fred Hutchinson Cancer Research Center, the University of Washington, and the Memorial Sloan-Kettering Cancer Center, all in the United States. It involved only ten people and was to test a new drug combination for a particularly malignant form of melanoma.

*It is important to find out what the **side effects** of treatments are. In the 2016 study, one patient developed vitiligo. This is a condition in which the skin loses its pigment, or color.*

The study tested an **immunotherapy** treatment. Immunotherapy encourages the body's **immune system** to find and kill cancer cells. Two types of drug treatments were tried, first separately, then as a combination. On their own, the drug treatments did not work, but when given together, the results were much better. Of the ten people in the study, two went into remission, which is when cancer disappears completely. Two patients had a small, but positive response to the treatment and three others remained the same. In another three, however, the disease progressed.

Although the study was small and the positive results l imited, all research like this helps scientists build their understanding of how cancer cells behave. It also adds to their knowledge of how certain drugs and treatments affect cancer. All studies of the disease can help beat it.

Studying the Enemy

Different cancers are caused by different types of cancerous cells. Knowing which type of cell a cancer starts in is vital to giving patients the correct treatment. Under a microscope, scientists study the structure of cancerous cells so they can tell which part of the body they come from.

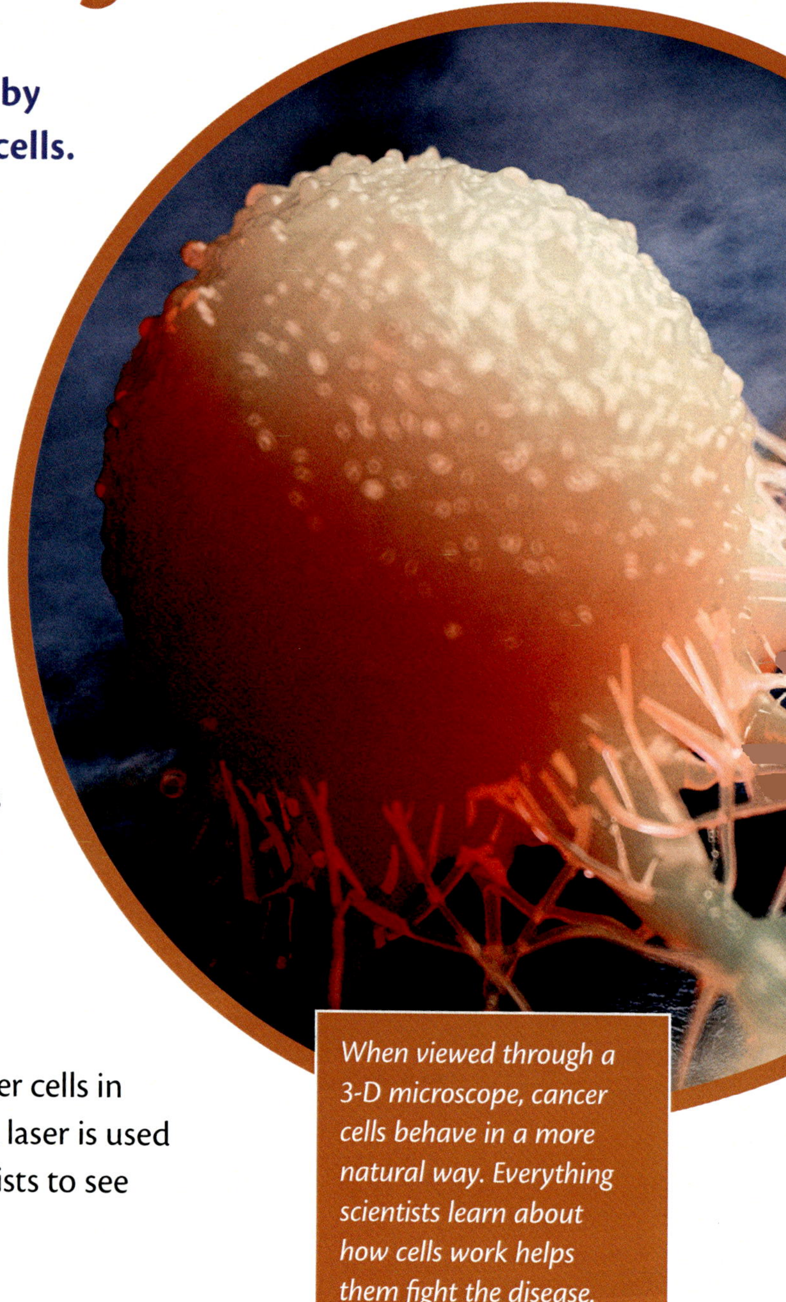

When viewed through a 3-D microscope, cancer cells behave in a more natural way. Everything scientists learn about how cells work helps them fight the disease.

Cancer in 3-D

With a traditional microscope, cells are viewed flat on a glass slide. This makes it difficult for scientists to judge how the cells behave in the body. However, when using a high-tech three-dimensional (3-D) microscope, scientists put the cancer cells in a substance called **collagen**. Then a laser is used to light up the cells, allowing scientists to see how they behave in the body.

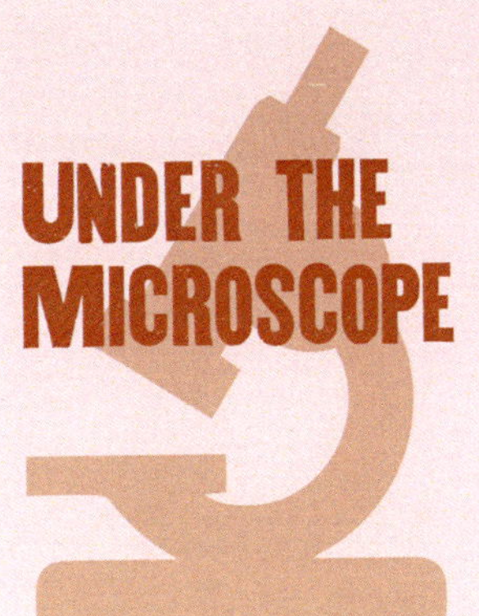

UNDER THE MICROSCOPE

A big advance in microscopy in recent years has been **fluorescence** microscopy. With this technique, scientists inject a dye into the patient's skin near the body area they suspect may have cancer cells. Two hours later, the scientists use a special camera to look inside the patient's body. The dye injected into the patient will have attached itself to any cancerous cells, showing them up clearly in a fluorescent color, which is picked up by the camera.

Under the Skin

In the past, to see if cells below the skin were damaged, doctors had to take a biopsy. Today, confocal microscopes can instead be used to **diagnose** skin cancers. These microscopes use a laser to scan the cells just beneath the skin. Using a confocal microscope is quicker and better for the patient, especially when examining skin on the face.

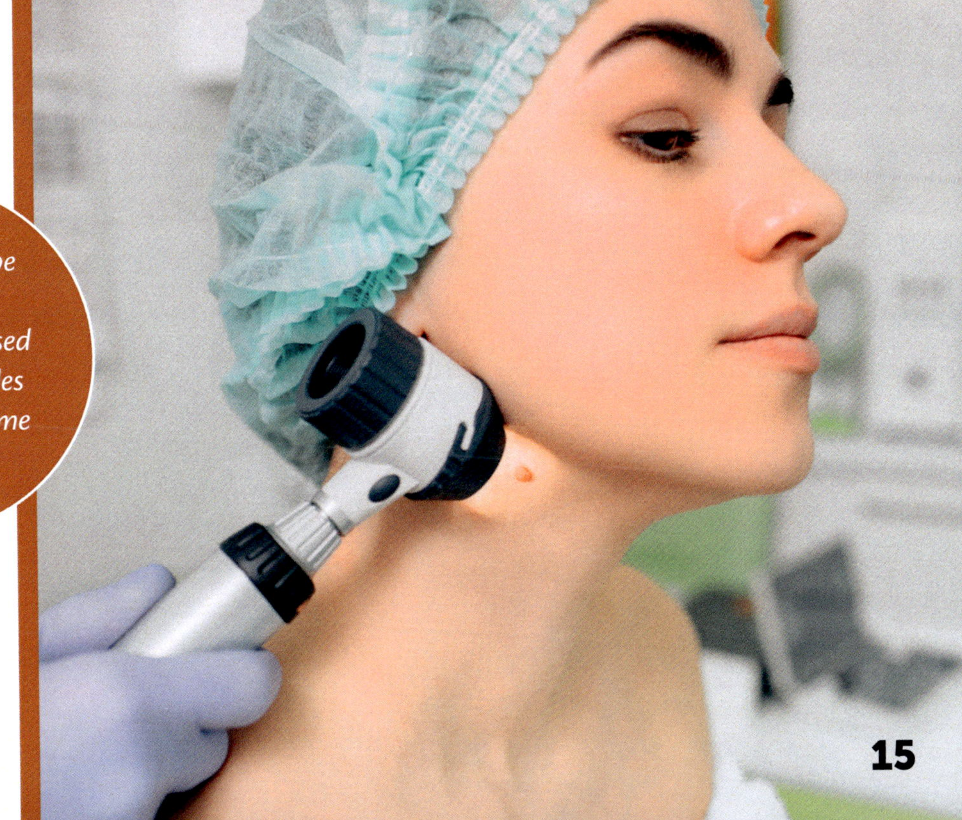

A dermatoscope is a handheld magnifier. It is used to examine moles that could become cancerous.

Armed with Medicine

Before cancer can be treated with medicine, it must be accurately diagnosed. There are several ways to do this. Usually, samples of blood, urine, or tissue are taken. These are then studied under a microscope to see if there are tumor markers. Tumor markers are substances produced by cancerous cells or other body cells when cancer is present in a person's body.

X-rays and Scans

Another way to diagnose cancer is to use imaging tests. Traditional X-rays can be used to diagnose cancers such as lung cancer. There are now also more sophisticated imaging tests that look inside the body to see if there is a tumor, what type it is, and how advanced it is.

Modern imaging tests include **computed tomography (CT) scans**, which take X-ray images of the inside of the body from different angles. Magnetic resonance imaging (MRI) scans create 3-D images of the inside of the body. Ultrasound scans use **high-frequency sound waves** that "bounce" off body parts to create images on a computer. **Positron emission tomography (PET) scans** and mammograms are two other types of imaging tests that are also used to find cancer. Mammograms are used to detect breast cancer only.

The person in this photograph is having a CT scan. Because people with cancer may not feel any symptoms, many countries have screening procedures, including CT scans, to find cancer. In these procedures, parts of the body that are at particular risk of developing cancer are checked for the disease.

Treating Tumors

Once diagnosed, how cancer is treated depends on the type of cancer. Surgery to remove a tumor was one of the earliest ways of dealing with cancer. Today, surgery is often used with other forms of therapy. Proton beam therapy is a type of **radiation therapy** that focuses in on the tumor, so there is less risk of damaging healthy surrounding tissue. This is especially important in treating tumors near to the spine and organs such as the liver.

Therapy Weapons

Some cancers are treated with different drug therapies. These include immunotherapy, chemotherapy, and **hormone** therapy. Chemotherapy uses drugs to kill cancerous cells. The drugs can be given to a patient by injection or as tablets. Once inside the body, the drugs seek out and destroy cancer cells.

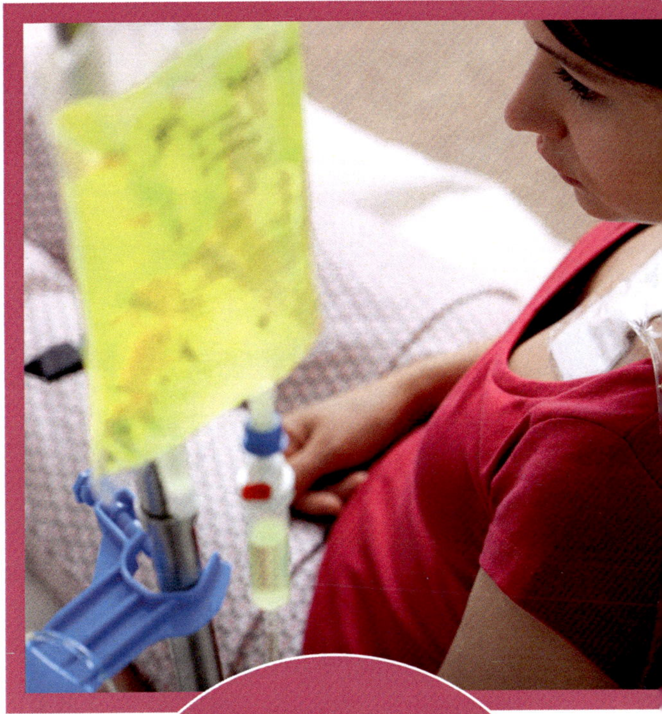

Traditional chemotherapy can be given to people as outpatients, which means that they do not have to stay in a hospital overnight. Special equipment is used to give patients the correct amount of drugs to fight their cancer.

"If we choose [treatments] wisely, we will be able to significantly increase the survival of many cancer patients and avoid subjecting others to unnecessary treatment."

Carsten Bokemeyer, cancer specialist, Hamburg, Germany

Vital Testing

Before cancer treatments can be rolled out for use on patients, they have to be carefully tested to make sure they work and do not have a lot of harmful side effects. One way that researchers do this is to run clinical trials.

Safety and Side Effects

Clinical trials are systems to test new drugs or treatments to see if they are safe. Under the supervision of experts, cancer patients are monitored on a regular basis to find out how their cancer is reacting to the drug being trialled. It is also important to find out if there are any side effects with the new drug, and how badly these affect patients. Side effects to drugs can be mild, such as headaches, to more severe, such as mood changes and weight loss.

Years of Testing

All patients who take part in a clinical trial must have chosen to do so—they give their consent, or agreement, to take part. Clinical trials often run for many years, until researchers are happy that the drugs are safe to use. Clinical trials can often involve thousands of people.

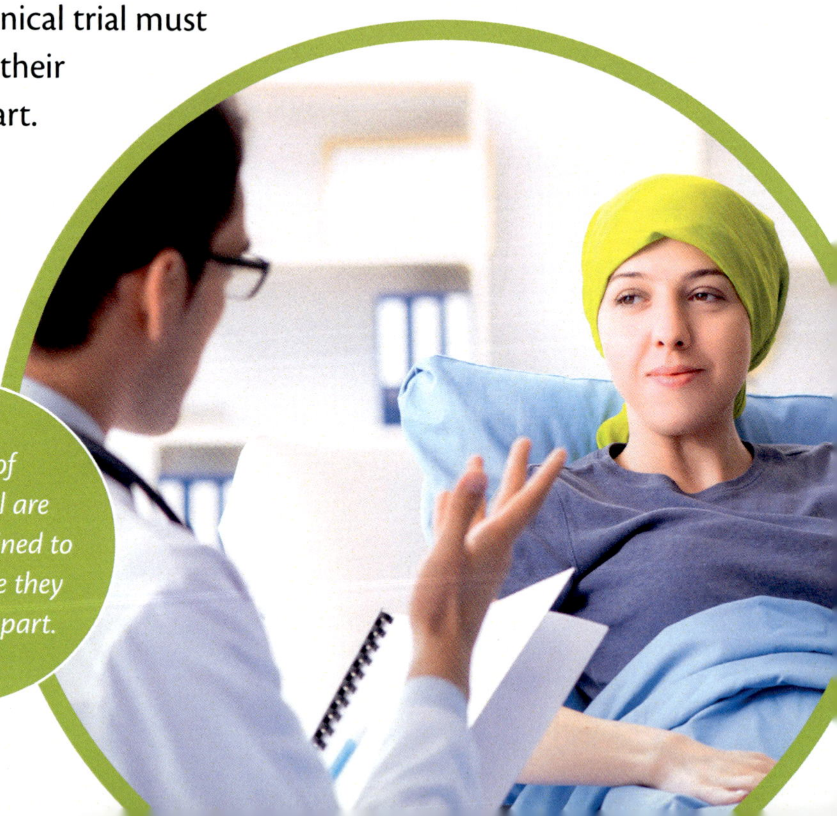

All parts of a clinical trial are carefully explained to patients before they agree to take part.

CASE STUDY: GROUNDBREAKING CANCER TRIAL

In 2013, a clinical trial was set up to test a new treatment for a rare form of childhood cancer called neuroblastoma. Neuroblastoma is formed from the cells that help a baby develop. When the baby is born, these cells normally vanish, but in some babies, the cells stay in the body and grow. This can lead to neuroblastoma. Many children are cured with drug treatments, but for a few, the cancer comes back.

Most people think that only adults get cancer, but it can also affect children and teenagers.

The trial is ongoing and taking place in the United Kingdom (U.K.) and across Europe. It involves 160 children.

The first aim of the trial is to test a specific combination of drugs to see how well it cures the cancer and what the side effects are. The second aim is to test a treatment that could prevent the cancer from recurring. The neuroblastoma cancer cells need a fresh supply of blood cells to keep them active, so the trial is testing a drug that can be used with chemotherapy to stop the blood vessels growing and feeding the cancer, without damaging any of the healthy tissue around the cells.

During the trial, blood and tumor samples are taken and tested to see how the cells are responding to the treatment. There is a long way to go with this trial, but if the outcome is positive, it will be a victory for science.

A Worldwide Fight

With advances in technology and medicine, deaths from cancer are starting to decrease. However, this trend is not happening in all countries around the world, especially in developing regions.

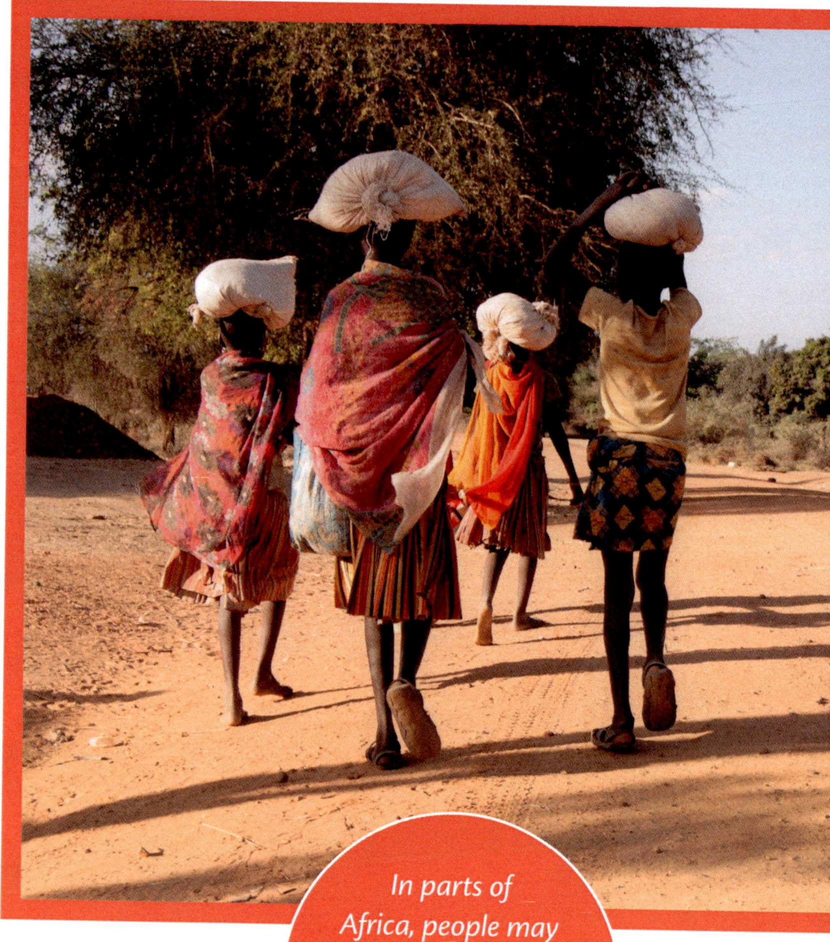

In parts of Africa, people may live far from big cities and have no access to a doctor or a hospital.

Cancer Cases Increasing

In developing regions, such as parts of India and Africa, deaths from cancer are, in fact, rising. In these regions, many people do not have access to the treatments that are more often available to people in developed countries. In some developing regions, hospitals in which people are treated for cancer and cancer-treating drugs are almost nonexistent. For example, radiation therapy is one of the most common ways to treat cancer but, of the 52 countries on the African continent, 29 are not able to offer this treatment.

Lifestyle Changes

It is expensive and takes time to persuade people to change lifestyle habits. In developed countries, such as the United Kingdom and the United States, there are ongoing campaigns supported by the governments and medical organizations encouraging people to exercise more, eat a healthier diet, and drink less alcohol. These are all lifestyle changes that can help reduce a person's chances of getting cancer. Developing regions tend to have more smokers and people who do not have a healthy diet, but governments in these countries cannot afford expensive public awareness campaigns to educate people about the dangers of smoking. People may also be unable to afford the types of food that can help keep them healthy.

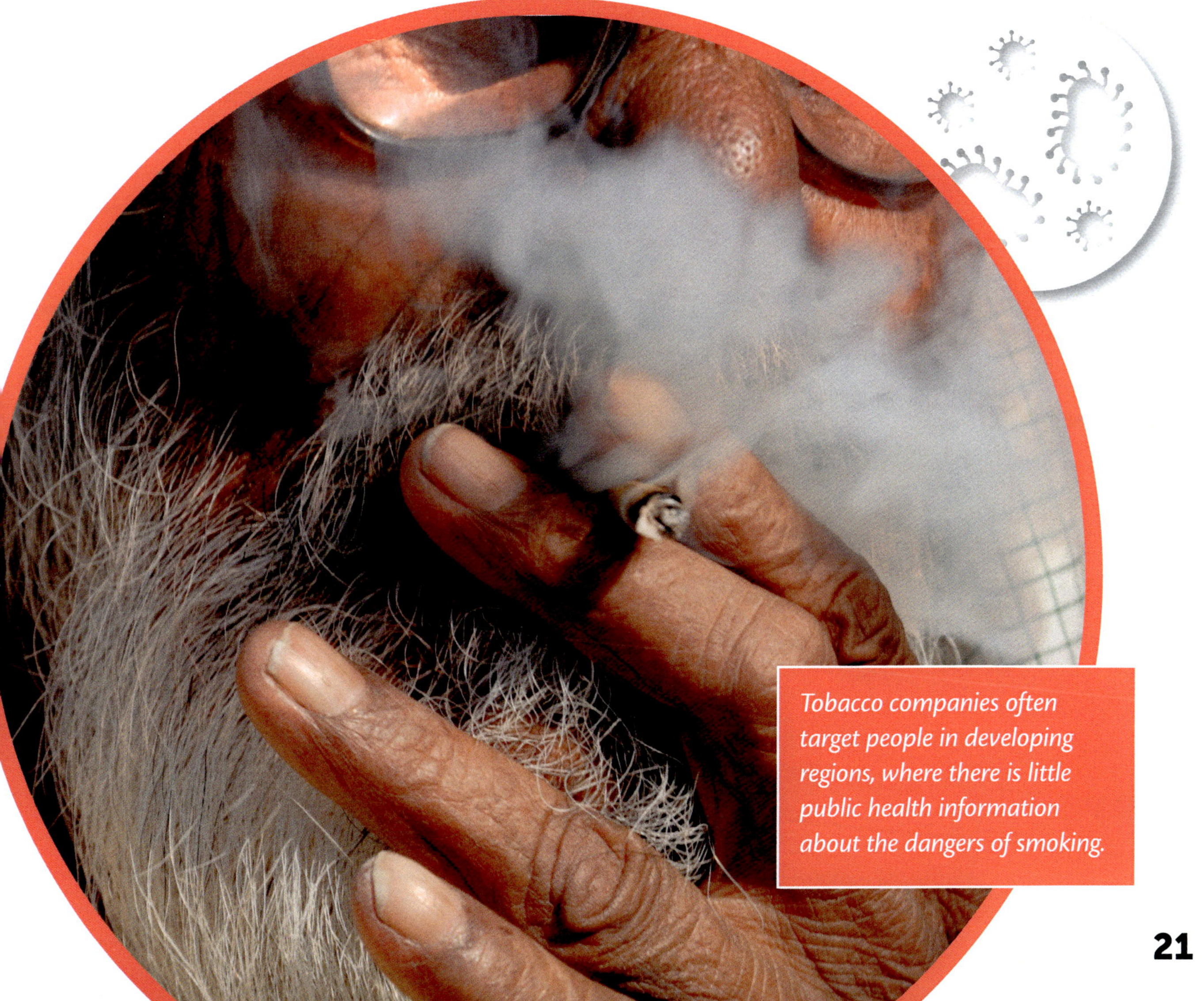

Tobacco companies often target people in developing regions, where there is little public health information about the dangers of smoking.

Enemy Education

Research has shown that in some countries there is a stigma around cancer. This means that people who have cancer view the disease as a disgrace or shame they have brought upon themselves and their families.

Hard-hitting health education is one way to help people change their lifestyles to prevent cancer.

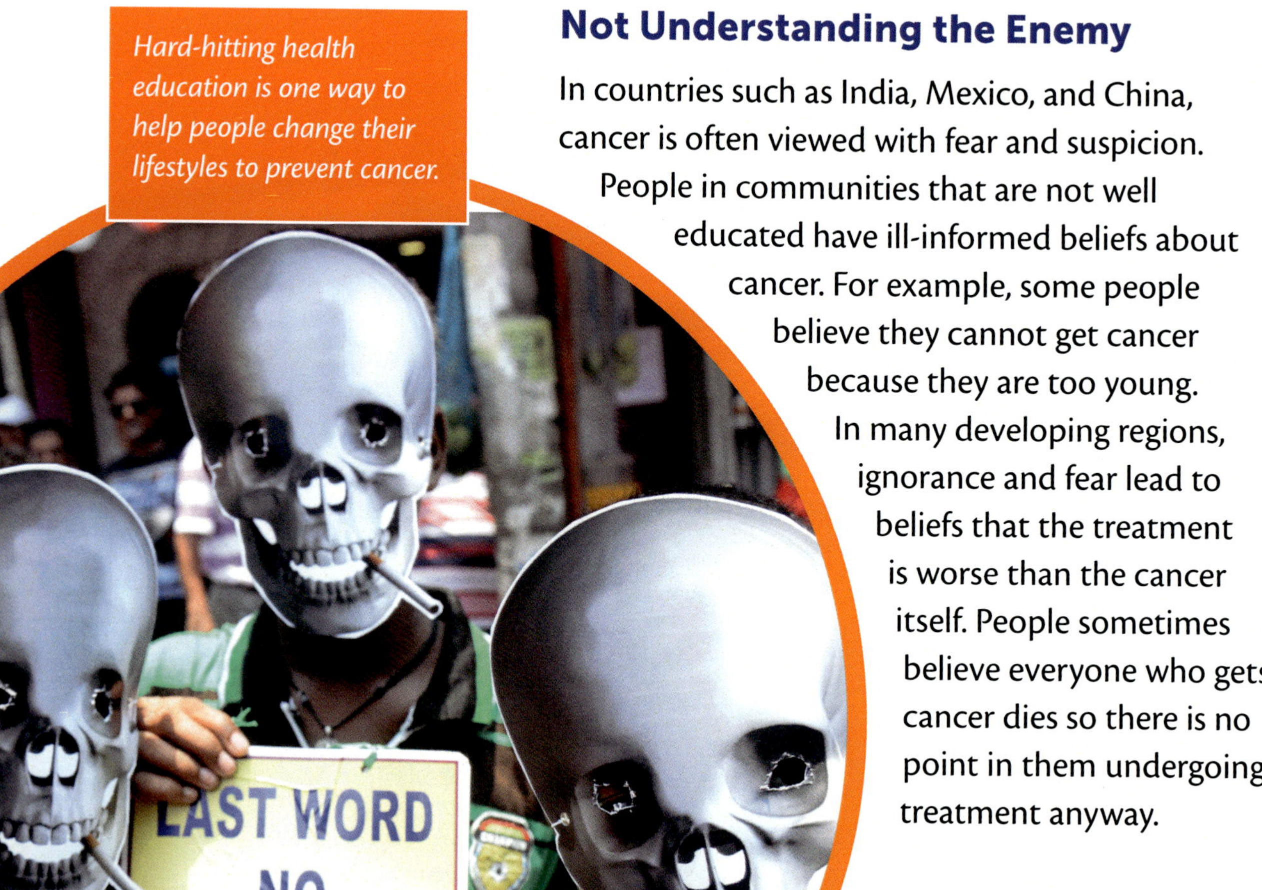

Not Understanding the Enemy

In countries such as India, Mexico, and China, cancer is often viewed with fear and suspicion. People in communities that are not well educated have ill-informed beliefs about cancer. For example, some people believe they cannot get cancer because they are too young. In many developing regions, ignorance and fear lead to beliefs that the treatment is worse than the cancer itself. People sometimes believe everyone who gets cancer dies so there is no point in them undergoing treatment anyway.

CASE STUDY: KNOWLEDGE IS POWER

Cancer cases are rising in India. There, education is the main weapon in the fight against the disease. The Indian Cancer Society (ICS) has a mission to increase awareness and knowledge about cancer. It hopes that this will lead to more people seeing doctors and getting an early diagnosis. This will lead to better treatment and to people improving their lifestyles, which in turn will lead to fewer cases of cancer.

In 2019, the ICS Cancer Awareness campaign included notices in newspapers in several Indian languages. They listed the signs of cancer, emphasized the importance of screening, and encouraged people to live a healthier lifestyle. The overall message was to not be scared of cancer.

The ICS also provides cancer **rehabilitation** centers where patients can learn new skills, such as clothes-making and printing. These activities keep people focused on something positive while they complete their treatment. The activities also give people a new skill that they can use after treatment and when they return to their communities.

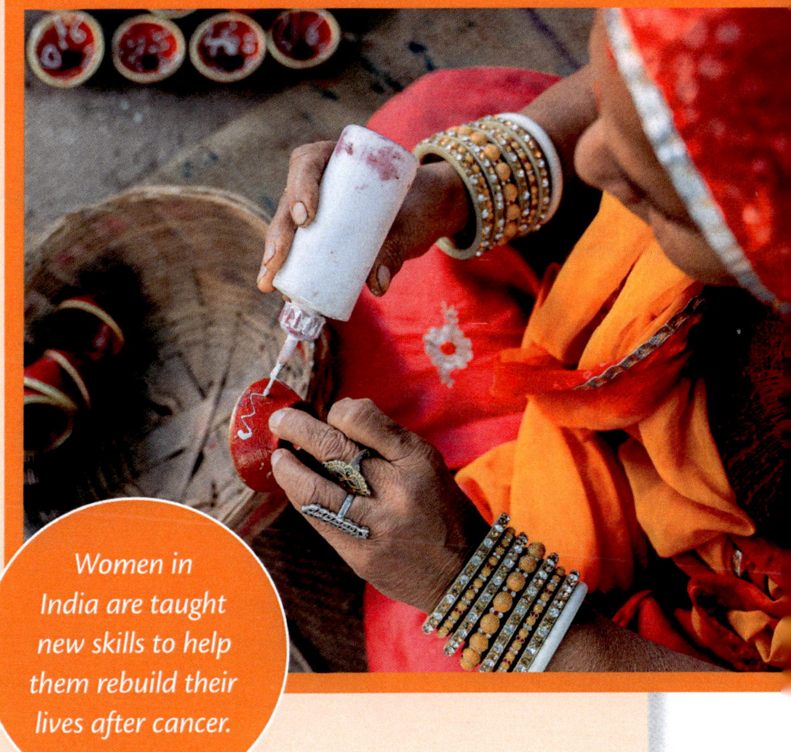

Women in India are taught new skills to help them rebuild their lives after cancer.

New Weapons

The battle against cancer is ongoing. Using advances in technology, science, and medicine, scientists now have the weapons to increase their understanding of cancer and beat the enemy.

Target the Cancer

A recent development in cancer treatment is precision medicine. This is the use of drugs based on the study of cancerous tissue from one individual. Scientists look at the DNA in the cancerous cells and search for any **genetic** changes that are causing the cancer to grow. Doctors can then prescribe drugs and other treatments that are specifically targeted at that person's cancer.

Scientists researching cancer can put their findings on a general ***database*** *that can be used by other scientists in their own country or worldwide.*

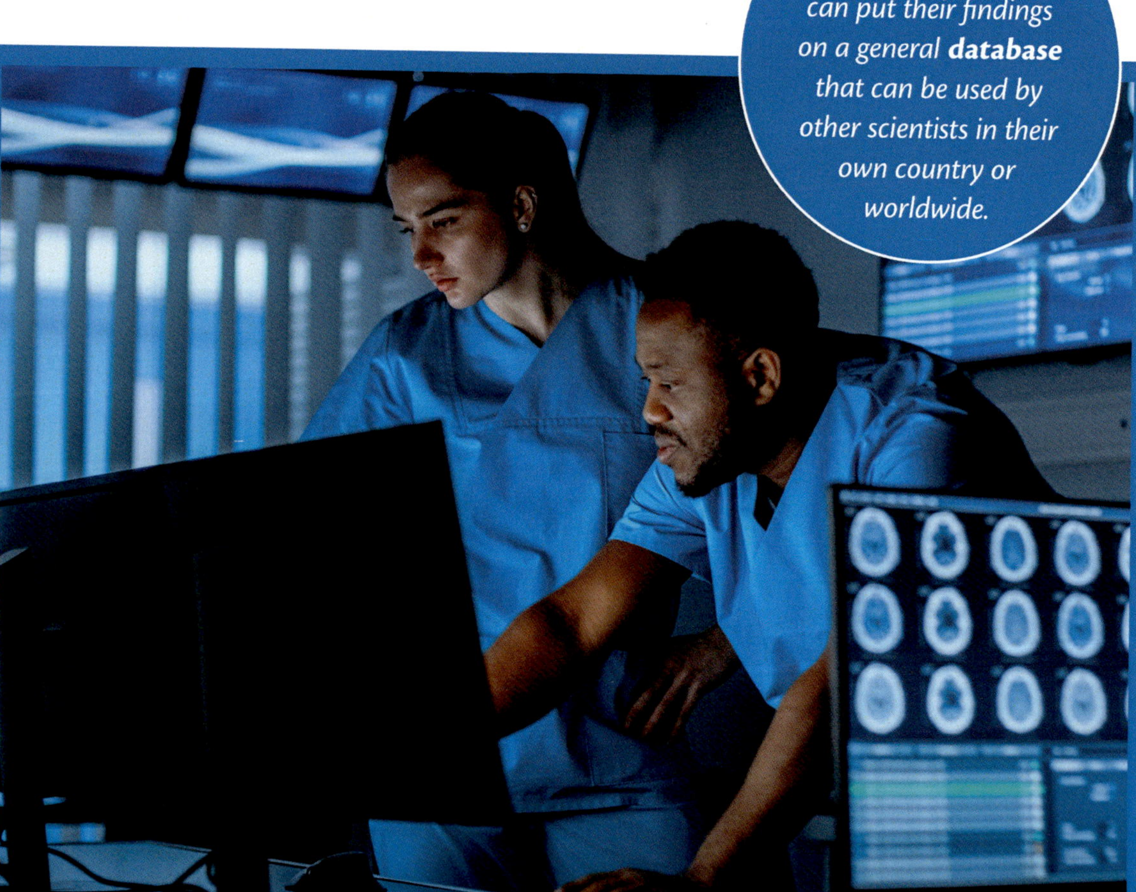

Outsmarting Cancer

The use of computing and **artificial intelligence (AI)** to help record and determine outcomes from clinical trials and forms of **data-based** research can help doctors predict the behavior of some types of cancers. For example, the National Cancer Institute (NCI) in Maryland and a team of researchers have collected more than 60,000 cervical images from an NCI clinical trial that began more than 25 years ago in an area in Costa Rica, Central America.

***Cervical** cells studied under a microscope help scientists learn more about which cells might be more likely to develop into cancer.*

Predicting the Future

The team observed any abnormalities in the images, then predicted whether they would lead to cancer. They kept health records of the women to see if their predictions were correct. With the development of AI, they created a computer algorithm, or code, to predict which women would develop cancer. The computer was twice as accurate as the doctors.

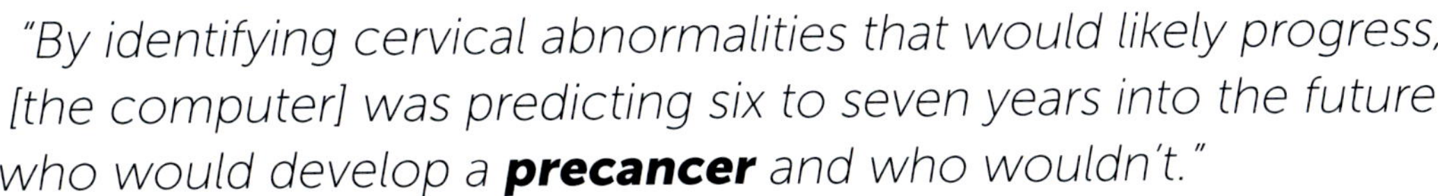

*"By identifying cervical abnormalities that would likely progress, [the computer] was predicting six to seven years into the future who would develop a **precancer** and who wouldn't."*

Mark Schiffman, NCI, Costa Rica

Future Warfare

These white blood cells have tracked down antigens and are destroying them. Cancer cells can be destroyed in the same way.

Many exciting developments are underway in cancer treatment. It is hoped that, used individually or in combination, these treatments will change the future of cancer warfare. Let's look at a few of them.

Kill the Cancer

Scientists are already using immunotherapy treatments for cancer. When the body is invaded by a harmful life form, called an antigen, the immune system recognizes the invading antigen and sends its white blood cells to attack it. In cancer patients, the immune system can be trained to attack, and then destroy, cancer cells in the same way.

A new and exciting development in immunotherapy is the creation of tailor-made cancer **vaccines**. The cancer cells in one person's tumor can be very different from the cancer cells in another person's tumor. For that reason, a vaccine designed to treat many different patients is not always effective—because it does not accurately target each person's particular type of cancer cells. However, if a patient is injected with a tailor-made vaccine that tells the immune system to recognize and destroy that person's particular cancer cells, it is far more likely to be effective.

Vaccines that use tumor cells from a patient's body can train the immune system to destroy any similar cancer cells that develop in the future.

Don't Eat Me!

A big problem with the immune system and cancer cells is that cancer cells can be sneaky! They are able to send out a "Don't eat me!" signal to the immune system so that, instead of destroying the cancer cells, it leaves them alone.

One way scientists are getting over this super-smart cancer trick is with **bacteria**. They program the bacteria to switch off the cancer cells' "Don't eat me!" message so that the immune system recognizes them as antigens, and destroys them. When scientists injected the bacteria into mice with cancer, they found that tumors within the mice shrank. They also discovered that further tumors were prevented from growing. It is hoped that the bacteria will be used in human cancer patients at some point in the future.

"The strongest weapon that we have to deal with any invasion in our body is our immune system."

Les Goldman, Senior Vice-President, Northwest Biotherapeutics

Timeline

Over the centuries, the diagnosis and treatment of cancer has changed enormously.

300s B.C.E. Greek physician Hippocrates is believed to identify malignant and benign tumors.

1500s Swiss physician Paracelsus recommends cancer be treated with the deadly substances mercury and arsenic.

1838 German physician Johannes Müller analyzes malignant and benign tumors under a microscope. He notes that cancer is formed in new cells in a diseased organ and that cancer can spread.

1850s German researcher Rudolf Virchow publishes a report on a patient whose body showed a high number of white blood cells. He named the condition leukemia.

1884 U.S. surgeon William Stewart Halsted introduces surgery to remove cancerous tumors in the breasts.

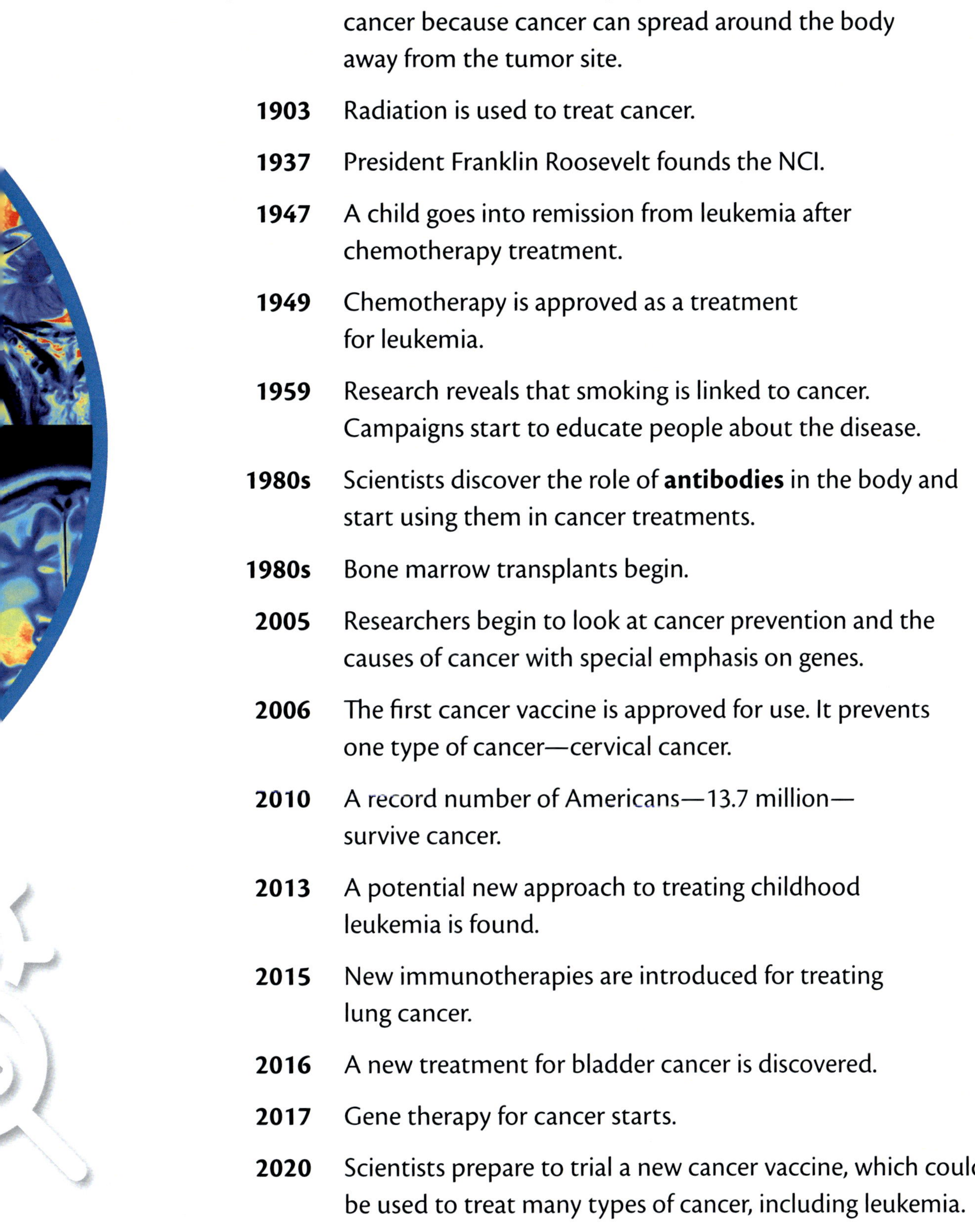

Early 1900s Research shows that surgery on its own does not cure cancer because cancer can spread around the body away from the tumor site.

1903 Radiation is used to treat cancer.

1937 President Franklin Roosevelt founds the NCI.

1947 A child goes into remission from leukemia after chemotherapy treatment.

1949 Chemotherapy is approved as a treatment for leukemia.

1959 Research reveals that smoking is linked to cancer. Campaigns start to educate people about the disease.

1980s Scientists discover the role of **antibodies** in the body and start using them in cancer treatments.

1980s Bone marrow transplants begin.

2005 Researchers begin to look at cancer prevention and the causes of cancer with special emphasis on genes.

2006 The first cancer vaccine is approved for use. It prevents one type of cancer—cervical cancer.

2010 A record number of Americans—13.7 million—survive cancer.

2013 A potential new approach to treating childhood leukemia is found.

2015 New immunotherapies are introduced for treating lung cancer.

2016 A new treatment for bladder cancer is discovered.

2017 Gene therapy for cancer starts.

2020 Scientists prepare to trial a new cancer vaccine, which could be used to treat many types of cancer, including leukemia.

Glossary

antibodies Substances produced by the body that fight off invading bacteria and viruses
artificial intelligence (AI) Computer programs that allow computers to problem-solve like humans
autopsies Surgical procedures that thoroughly examine a corpse to figure out the cause of death and the extent of a disease
bacteria Microscopic living things that can cause infection and sickness
bowel A part of the body in which digestive processes take place
cellular Relating to cells
cervical To do with the cervix, part of a woman's reproductive system
collagen A substance found in human tissue
computed tomography (CT) scans X-ray images made with the help of multiple X-ray measurements and a computer
database Relying on observation and experiments
data-based Working with facts and statistics
deoxyribonucleic acid (DNA) A part of the body's cells that gives each individual their own unique characteristics
developing regions Areas where the population may lack access to jobs, food, water, education, health care, and housing
diagnose To confirm a person has an illness
fluorescence Light absorbed by a substance then re-emitted
genes Parts of DNA that are passed down through a family
genetic Related to genes
high-frequency sound waves Sound waves that produce sounds too high-pitched for humans to hear
hormone A substance in the body that controls certain bodily functions
immune system The parts of the body that work together to protect it against sickness
immunotherapy A type of cancer treatment that helps the immune system fight cancer
laser A powerful beam of light
microscopes Devices that magnify, or make bigger, tiny objects that can otherwise not be seen with the naked eye
moles Dark brown or black marks on the skin that are usually harmless but can become cancerous
organs Parts of the body, such as the heart or lungs, that have specific functions
physicist A person who studies the nature of matter and energy
positron emission tomography (PET) scans Medical examinations in which substances are injected into the body that then reveal cancerous cells
precancer Abnormal cells that could turn into cancerous cells
radiation therapy Using high-energy radiation to kill cancer cells and shrink tumors
rehabilitation Help given to those who want to go back to their normal way of life after a long or severe illness and treatment
side effects Unpleasant effects that taking a certain drug has on a person, such as making them feel dizzy
tissue A group of cells of the same type, such as muscle cells, that perform a job together
tumor An abnormal mass of tissue
ultraviolet (UV) A type of sunlight that can lead to skin cancer
vaccines Substance that help protect against certain diseases
white blood cells Cells that attack and destroy enemy invaders, such as bacteria

Learning More

Find out more about cancer and how the war against this deadly disease is being won.

Books

Olsher, Sara S. *Cancer Party!* Mighty + Bright, 2019.

Shea, John. *Viruses Up Close* (Under the Microscope). Gareth Stevens, 2013.

Simons, Rae. *A Kid's Guide to Cancer* (Understanding Disease and Wellness: Kids' Guides to Why People Get Sick and How They Can Stay Well). Village Earth Press, 2016.

Wood, John. *Bacteria in Our World* (Under the Microscope). KidHaven Publishing, 2019.

Websites

Learn about cancer, what it is, how it is diagnosed, and how it can be treated at:
https://kidshealth.org/en/kids/cancer.html

Discover more about the world of cells, what they do, how they behave, and why they are important at:
https://kids.kiddle.co/Cell

Read inspiring stories about children from around the world who have developed cancer and how they and their families have dealt with it at:
www.worldchildcancer.org

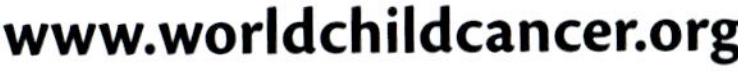

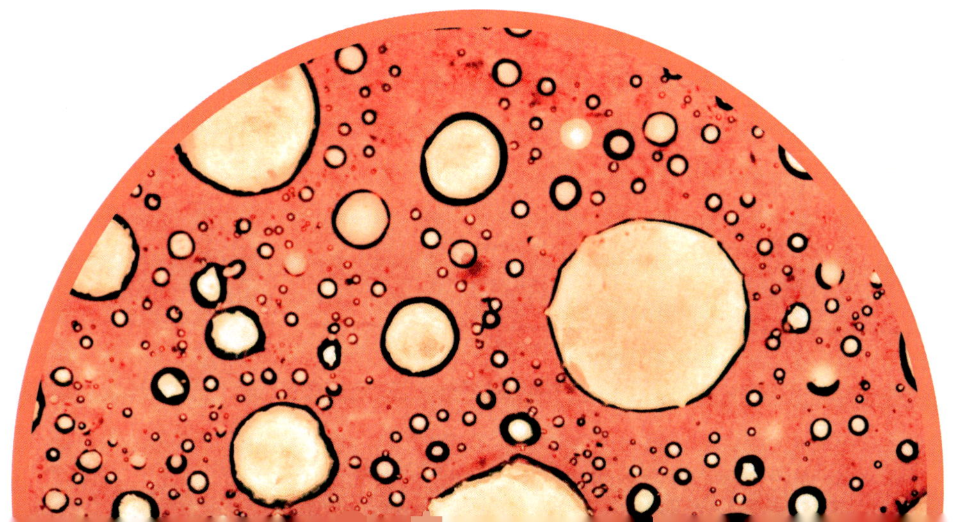

Index

antibodies 29
artificial intelligence (AI) 25

bacteria 27
benign tumors 9, 28
breast cancer 4, 9, 16, 28

cell division 8, 9
cell theory 6
cervical cancer 25, 29
chemotherapy 17, 19, 29
clinical trials 18, 19, 25
computed tomography (CT) scans 16

deoxyribonucleic acid (DNA) 8, 24

education 12, 21, 22, 23, 29

genes 8, 24, 29

Hooke, Robert 5, 6
hormone therapy 17

immunotherapy 13, 17, 26

Janssen, Hans and Zacharias 5

leukemia 7, 10, 11, 28, 29
lung cancer 4, 10, 16, 29

magnetic resonance imaging (MRI) scans 16
malignant melanoma 13
malignant tumors 9, 28
mammograms 16
microscopes 4, 5, 6, 7, 9, 14, 15, 16, 25, 28

neuroblastoma 19

positron emission tomography (PET) scans 16

radiation therapy 17, 20

skin cancer 4, 11, 12, 13, 15
smoking 21, 29
stigma 22
studies 13
surgery 17, 28, 29
symptoms 8, 10, 11, 16

tumors 9, 10, 16, 17, 19, 26, 27, 28, 29

ultrasound scans 16

vaccines 26, 27, 29
Virchow, Rudolf 6, 7, 28

white blood cells 7, 10, 26, 28

X-rays 10, 16

ABOUT THE AUTHOR

Sarah Eason has written many science books for children, from space to biology. She particularly loves finding out how our complicated and fascinating human bodies work.